Discover

Wall Pilates

A Beginner's Guide

to Core Strength

and Flexibility for Women Over Fifty

By Jessica Peters

Discover Wall Pilates
A Beginner's Guide to Core Strength and Flexibility
for Women Over Fifty

In association with:
Biz Social Marketing Agency
63 East 11400 South
Suite #230
Sandy, UT 84070
BizSocialMarketing.com

ISBN: 979-8-8693-4835-7 (Paperback)
ISBN: 979-8-8693-4836-4 (eBook)

Disclaimer

The content provided in this book, "Discover Wall Pilates" is intended for informational and educational purposes only. While wall Pilates can offer numerous benefits for physical, mental, and emotional well-being, it is essential to consult with a qualified healthcare professional before beginning any new exercise program, especially if you have pre-existing health conditions or concerns.

The information presented in this book is not intended to diagnose, treat, cure, or prevent any disease or medical condition. It should not be used as a substitute for professional medical advice, diagnosis, or treatment. Always seek the advice of your physician or other qualified healthcare provider with any questions you may have regarding your health or a medical condition.

Individual results from wall Pilates may vary depending on age, fitness level, medical history, and adherence to the recommended exercises and guidelines. It is essential to listen to your body and modify or discontinue any exercise that causes discomfort or pain.

By engaging in the practices outlined in this book, you acknowledge and accept full responsibility for your health and well-being. The author and publisher of this book disclaim any liability for any injury, loss, or damage incurred as a result of the use or misuse of the information provided.

Remember, wall Pilates is a journey of self-discovery and transformation, and it is essential to approach it with mindfulness, patience, and compassion for yourself. Always prioritize your safety and well-being above all else.

Individual results may vary.

Table of Contents

Introduction

Hello, beautiful souls! Welcome to the world of Wall Pilates – where strength meets serenity, and transformation begins from the inside out. I'm thrilled to take you on this journey, guiding you through the empowering practice of Wall Pilates, a revolutionary approach to fitness that I'm passionate about sharing.

As someone who has embraced holistic wellness for many years, I've seen firsthand the profound impact that mindful movement can have on our bodies and spirits. As a health advocate, I've explored various fitness modalities, always searching for the perfect balance of strength, flexibility, and inner peace.

When I discovered Wall Pilates, it was like finding the missing piece of the puzzle. It's not just a workout – it's a way of life. With its gentle yet effective techniques, Wall Pilates has helped me sculpt my body, ease my mind, and tap into a deeper connection with myself.

In this book, I'll be your guide as we dive into the world of Wall Pilates together. We'll explore the fundamentals of this transformative practice, learn essential techniques for alignment and engagement, and discover a treasure trove of beginner-friendly exercises to kickstart your journey to vibrant health and vitality.

But more than just a fitness regimen, Wall Pilates is a mindset – a philosophy of living with intention and grace. It's about embracing your body's innate wisdom, honoring its strengths and limitations, and nurturing yourself with kindness and compassion every step of the way.

So, get ready to awaken your inner powerhouse, ignite your passion for movement, and unleash your radiant energy with Wall Pilates. It's time to step into your power, embrace your potential, and shine brighter than ever before. Together, let's make every moment a masterpiece. Welcome to the transformative world of Wall Pilates – where miracles happen, one breath at a time.

Jessica Peters

14

Chapter 1

Discovering the Magic of Wall Pilates

Well, hello there, gorgeous! Are you ready to dive headfirst into the enchanting world of Wall Pilates? Buckle up, because I'm about to take you on a journey that will leave you feeling stronger, sexier, and more alive than ever before!

Now, let me tell you, when I first stumbled upon Wall Pilates, I was absolutely floored. It was like stumbling upon a hidden treasure – a secret oasis of strength, flexibility, and inner peace just waiting to be discovered.

But what exactly is Wall Pilates, you ask? Oh, honey, let me break it down for you. Picture this: you're standing tall, back against the wall, feeling the support of its sturdy embrace as you move through a series of graceful, empowering exercises. With each breath, each movement, you can feel your body coming alive, your muscles awakening, and your spirit soaring to new heights.

But here's the best part – Wall Pilates isn't just about building a killer bod (although, let's be real, that's definitely a perk!). It's about tapping into your inner strength, reconnecting with your body, and embracing your power like never before. It's about saying "hell yes" to life, owning your worth, and strutting through the world with confidence and grace.

So, my dear, get ready to unleash your inner goddess, because with Wall Pilates by your side, the sky's the limit. Are you ready to discover the magic of Wall Pilates and unleash your full potential? Well, darling, let's do this – together!

Chapter 2

Creating Your Sacred Space for Wall Pilates Bliss

Hello there, darlings! Are you ready to transform your home into a sanctuary of serenity and strength? In this chapter, we're going to dive deep into the art of creating your very own sacred space for Wall Pilates bliss.

Creating a space where you can escape the chaos of the outside world and dive deep into your practice is absolutely essential. So, grab your favorite scented candles, dim the lights, and let's get started!

First things first – let's talk about selecting the perfect wall for your Wall Pilates practice. You want a wall that's sturdy, supportive, and free from distractions. Whether it's a blank canvas in your living room or a quiet corner in your bedroom, find a space that speaks to your soul and makes you feel grounded and centered.

Next up, let's talk equipment. Now, you don't need a ton of fancy gadgets to get started with Wall Pilates. All you really need is a sturdy yoga mat, a couple of yoga blocks, and maybe a resistance band or two to add a little extra oomph to your practice.

Once you've got your space set up and your equipment in place, it's time to set the mood. Dim the lights, put on some soothing music, and let yourself sink into the present moment. This is your time to escape, to unwind, and to reconnect with yourself on a deeper level.

So, my dear, are you ready to transform your home into a haven of peace and tranquility? Are you ready to create your very own sacred space for Wall Pilates bliss? Well, darling, let's roll out that mat, strike a pose, and let the magic unfold. Your journey to inner strength and outer radiance starts right here, right now. Let's do this!

Chapter 3

Mastering the Fundamentals of Wall Pilates

Well, hello there, fabulous friends! Are you ready to dive deep into the heart of Wall Pilates and unlock the secrets of strength, stability, and serenity? Because in this chapter, we're going to master the fundamentals of Wall Pilates like never before.

Now, I know what you're thinking – mastering the fundamentals sounds a little intimidating, right? But trust me, darling, it's easier than you think. It's all about finding your center, tuning into your breath, and embracing the beauty of each and every movement.

So, let's start with the breath, shall we? Take a deep breath in through your nose, feeling your belly rise as you fill your lungs with fresh, invigorating air. And now, exhale slowly through your mouth, releasing any tension or stress that's been weighing you down. Ah, doesn't that feel better already?

Next up, let's talk alignment. When it comes to Wall Pilates, proper alignment is absolutely key. Stand tall, shoulders back, core engaged, and imagine a string pulling you up towards the sky. Feel the support of the wall against your back, grounding you and anchoring you in the present moment.

Now, let's move into the exercises. Start with something simple – maybe a gentle twist or a pelvic tilt

– and really focus on connecting with your body. Feel the muscles engage, the energy flow, and the tension melt away with each and every movement.

And remember, darling, there's no rush. Take your time, listen to your body, and honor its wisdom. Wall Pilates is a journey, not a destination, and every step along the way is a chance to grow, to learn, and to embrace your inner strength like never before.

So, are you ready to master the fundamentals of Wall Pilates and unleash your full potential? Are you ready to stand tall, breathe deep, and move with grace and ease? Well, my dear, let's dive in and discover the magic together. Your body, mind, and spirit will thank you for it. Let's do this!

Jessica Peters

Chapter 4

Embracing Beginner-Friendly Wall Pilates Exercises

Well, hello there, fabulous souls! Are you ready to ignite your passion for movement and unleash your inner powerhouse with a collection of beginner-friendly Wall Pilates exercises? In this chapter, we're going to dive headfirst into a world of grace, strength, and empowerment like never before.

Now, I know what you're thinking – beginner-friendly exercises? That sounds like my kind of jam! And let me tell you, darling, you're in for a treat. These exercises may be gentle, but they pack a powerful punch when it comes to sculpting your body, toning your muscles, and unleashing your radiant energy.

So, let's start with something simple – maybe a gentle wall squat or a supported plank. Feel the support of the wall against your back, grounding you and anchoring you in the present moment. Engage your core, lengthen your spine, and let yourself sink into the movement with grace and ease.

Next up, let's explore some gentle stretches to release tension, improve flexibility, and enhance your overall range of motion. From soothing shoulder rolls to invigorating chest openers, each stretch is designed to nurture your body and soul with love and compassion.

And remember, darling, there's no such thing as perfection in Wall

Pilates. It's all about progress, not perfection. So, take your time, listen to your body, and honor its wisdom. Whether you're a seasoned pro or a total newbie, there's always something new to learn, something new to discover, and something new to embrace.

So, are you ready to embrace beginner-friendly Wall Pilates exercises and unleash your full potential? Are you ready to step into your power, own your worth, and shine brighter than ever before? Well, my dear, let's roll out that mat, strike a pose, and let the magic unfold. Your body, mind, and spirit will thank you for it. Let's do this!

Jessica Peters

34

Chapter 5

Cultivating Strength and Stability with Wall Pilates

Alright, my beautiful friends, are you ready to tap into your inner warrior and build strength and stability from the inside out? Because in this chapter, we're going to explore a series of empowering Wall Pilates exercises designed to sculpt your body, tone your muscles, and enhance your overall stability and balance.

Now, I want you to imagine yourself standing tall, back against the wall, feeling the support of its sturdy embrace as you move through each exercise with grace and determination. Engage your core, lengthen your spine, and let yourself sink into the movement with power and purpose.

Let's start with something simple – maybe a wall push-up or a standing leg lift. Feel the muscles engage, the energy flow, and the tension melt away with each and every movement. And remember, darling, it's not about how many reps you can do or how long you can hold a pose. It's about connecting with your body, listening to its wisdom, and honoring its needs with love and compassion.

So, whether you're working on sculpting those arms, toning those legs, or strengthening that core, there's a Wall Pilates exercise for you. And with each movement, each breath, you'll feel yourself growing stronger, more resilient, and more radiant than ever before.

So, are you ready to unleash your inner warrior and embrace the power of strength and stability with Wall Pilates? Well, my dear, let's roll out that mat, strike a pose, and let the magic unfold. Your body, mind, and spirit will thank you for it. Let's do this!

Chapter 6

Nurturing Flexibility and Freedom of Movement

Hello, hello, my beautiful souls! Are you ready to embrace the transformative power of flexibility and freedom of movement? Because in this chapter, we're going to explore a series of gentle, yet effective Wall Pilates stretches designed to release tension, improve flexibility, and enhance your overall range of motion.

Now, I want you to picture yourself standing tall, back against the wall, feeling the support of its sturdy embrace as you sink into each stretch with grace and ease. Take a deep breath in, and as you exhale, let yourself melt deeper into the stretch, feeling the tension melt away and the energy flow freely throughout your body.

Let's start with something simple – maybe a gentle shoulder stretch or a relaxing hamstring stretch. Feel the muscles lengthen, the joints open, and the spirit soar with each and every movement. And remember, darling, it's not about forcing your body into a pretzel-like shape or pushing yourself beyond your limits. It's about honoring your body's needs, listening to its wisdom, and nurturing it with love and compassion.

So, whether you're working on releasing tension in your neck and shoulders, improving flexibility in your hips and hamstrings, or finding greater freedom of movement in your spine, there's a Wall Pilates stretch for you. And with each stretch, each breath, you'll feel yourself becoming more open, more supple, and more alive than ever before.

So, are you ready to embrace the power of flexibility and freedom of movement with Wall Pilates? Well, my dear, let's roll out that mat, strike a pose, and let the magic unfold. Your body, mind, and spirit will thank you for it. Let's do this!

Jessica Peters

44

Chapter 7

Harnessing the Mind-Body Connection in Wall Pilates

Well, hello there, beautiful souls! Are you ready to tap into the profound wisdom of your body and harness the transformative power of the mind-body connection? Because in this chapter, we're going to explore the art of mindfulness in Wall Pilates practice, teaching you how to cultivate presence, awareness, and self-love with each breath and movement.

Now, I want you to imagine yourself standing tall, back against the wall, feeling the support of its sturdy embrace as you move through each exercise with grace and intention. Take a deep breath in, and as you exhale, let yourself sink deeper into the present moment, feeling the tension melt away and the energy flow freely throughout your body.

Let's start with something simple – maybe a mindful breathing exercise or a gentle body scan. Feel the breath fill your lungs, the sensations arise, and the mind settle into a state of calm and clarity. And remember, darling, it's not about clearing your mind of all thoughts or achieving some elusive state of perfection. It's about being present, being aware, and being kind to yourself in each and every moment.

So, whether you're working on cultivating mindfulness in your movement, practicing gratitude for your body and its capabilities, or simply taking a moment to pause and breathe, there's a mindfulness practice for you. And with each breath, each movement, you'll feel yourself becoming more grounded, more centered, and more alive than ever before.

So, are you ready to embrace the power of the mind-body connection with Wall Pilates? Well, my dear, let's roll out that mat, strike a pose, and let the magic unfold. Your body, mind, and spirit will thank you for it. Let's do this!

Jessica Peters

50

Chapter 8

Embracing Self-Care and Self-Love on Your Wall Pilates Journey

Hey there, beautiful souls! Are you ready to embark on a journey of self-discovery and self-love like never before? Because in this chapter, we're going to explore the importance of self-care and self-love on your Wall Pilates journey, teaching you how to nurture your body, mind, and spirit with kindness, compassion, and grace.

Now, I want you to take a moment to pause, to breathe, and to connect with yourself on a deeper level. Close your eyes, place your hand over your heart, and feel the gentle rhythm of your breath as it flows in and out of your body. This is your time, your space, and your opportunity to honor yourself with love and reverence.

Let's start by talking about self-care. What does it mean to you? Maybe it's taking a long, luxurious bath after a challenging workout. Maybe it's curling up with a good book and a cup of tea on a rainy day. Or maybe it's simply taking a few moments each day to check in with yourself, to listen to your body's needs, and to honor its wisdom with compassion and grace.

Next up, let's talk about self-love. How do you show yourself love and appreciation on a daily basis? Maybe it's through positive affirmations, reminding yourself of your worth and value. Maybe it's through acts of kindness, both towards yourself and others. Or maybe it's simply through embracing your flaws, imperfections, and quirks with love and acceptance.

So, whether you're practicing self-care through nourishing movement, healthy nutrition, or restful sleep, or showing yourself love through positive self-talk, acts of kindness, or self-compassion, there's no right or wrong way to do it. It's all about finding what works for you, what fills your cup, and what brings you joy and fulfillment.

So, are you ready to embrace self-care and self-love on your Wall Pilates journey? Well, my dear, let's roll out that mat, strike a pose, and let the magic unfold. Your body, mind, and spirit will thank you for it. Let's do this!

Jessica Peters

56

Chapter 9

Embracing the Power of Mindfulness in Wall Pilates Practice

Hey there, gorgeous souls! Are you ready to tap into the profound wisdom of your body and harness the transformative power of mindfulness like never before? Because in this chapter, we're going to explore the art of mindfulness in Wall Pilates practice, teaching you how to cultivate presence, awareness, and self-love with each breath and movement.

Now, I want you to take a moment to pause, to breathe, and to connect with yourself on a deeper level. Close your eyes, soften your gaze, and feel the gentle rhythm of your breath as it flows in and out of your body. This is your time, your space, and your opportunity to anchor yourself in the present moment and to embrace the beauty of each and every sensation.

Let's start by talking about mindfulness. What does it mean to you? Maybe it's about being fully present in the here and now, letting go of worries about the past or future. Maybe it's about cultivating a sense of curiosity and openness, approaching each moment with fresh eyes and an open heart. Or maybe it's simply about being kind to yourself, embracing whatever thoughts, feelings, or sensations arise with love and acceptance.

Next up, let's talk about incorporating mindfulness into

your Wall Pilates practice. How can you bring more mindfulness into your movement, your breath, and your overall approach to fitness? Maybe it's about focusing on the sensations in your body as you move through each exercise, tuning into the subtle nuances of your alignment, engagement, and energy. Maybe it's about using your breath as an anchor, a reminder to stay present and engaged with each moment as it unfolds. Or maybe it's simply about approaching your practice with a sense of curiosity, openness, and non-judgment, embracing whatever arises with love and compassion.

So, whether you're practicing mindfulness through breathwork, body awareness, or simply being present in the moment, there's no right or wrong way to do it. It's all about finding what works for you, what resonates with you, and what brings you joy and fulfillment.

So, are you ready to embrace the power of mindfulness in your Wall Pilates practice? Well, my dear, let's roll out that mat, strike a pose, and let the magic unfold. Your body, mind, and spirit will thank you for it. Let's do this!

Chapter 10

Celebrating Your Journey with Wall Pilates

Hey there, beautiful souls! Can you believe it? You've reached the final chapter of your transformative journey with Wall Pilates, and let me tell you, my heart is bursting with pride and joy. So, let's take a moment to celebrate all that you've accomplished, all that you've overcome, and all that you've become on this incredible journey of self-discovery and empowerment.

Now, I want you to close your eyes, take a deep breath in, and let yourself bask in the glow of your own radiant light. Feel the warmth of your heart, the strength of your spirit, and the beauty of your soul shining brightly from within. This is your moment, your time to shine, and your opportunity to honor yourself with love and reverence.

Let's start by celebrating your achievements. Maybe you've discovered newfound strength and flexibility in your body, mastering challenging exercises that once seemed impossible. Maybe you've found a deeper sense of peace and serenity in your mind, cultivating mindfulness and presence in each moment. Or maybe you've simply embraced the journey, showing up for yourself day after day, with courage, determination, and grace.

Next up, let's talk about gratitude. What are you grateful for on this journey? Maybe it's the support of loved ones who have cheered you on every step of the way. Maybe it's the resilience of your body, which has carried you through every challenge and triumph with grace and strength. Or maybe it's simply the gift of this moment, this opportunity to connect with yourself, to embrace your power, and to shine your light brightly for all the world to see.

So, whether you're celebrating your achievements, expressing gratitude for your blessings, or simply reveling in the joy of this moment, know that you are loved, you are cherished, and you are worthy of all the happiness and success in the world.

So, my dear, let's raise a glass, toast to your brilliance, and celebrate the incredible journey you've taken with Wall Pilates. Your body, mind, and spirit will thank you for it. Cheers to you, my beautiful friend. May your light shine brightly for all eternity. Let's do this!

Jessica Peters

Bonus Chapter

10 Beginner Wall Pilates Exercises with Pictures

Here are ten absolutely beginner-friendly wall Pilates exercises that I just adore! Each one comes with its own fabulous benefits and easy-to-follow instructions:

1. Wall Roll Down

Benefits: Enhances spinal flexibility and engages core muscles.

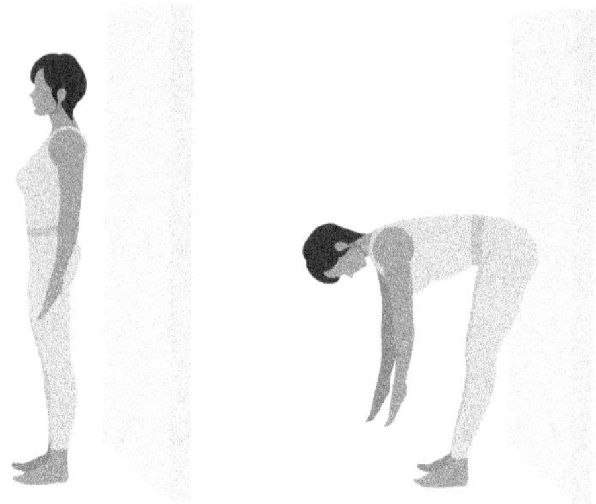

How to Do It: Stand with your back against the wall, feet slightly away from the base. Slowly roll down the wall, vertebra by vertebra, until your lower back is also touching the wall. Tuck your chin slightly and roll back up to the starting position. Hold up to 30 seconds. Rest 30-60 seconds and repeat three times.

2. Wall Squats

Benefits: Strengthens legs, buttocks, and core.

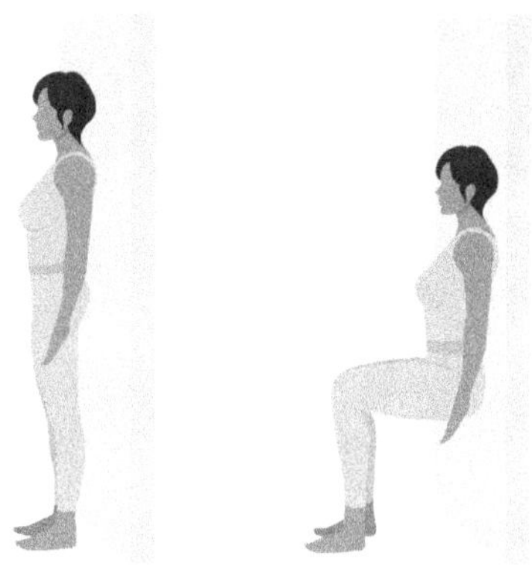

How to Do It: Stand with your back against the wall, feet about hip-width apart. Slide down the wall into a squat position, making sure your knees are aligned with your ankles. Press your back into the wall and engage your quads, glutes, and hamstrings to stay steady. Hold anywhere from 10 to 60 seconds. Rest 30-60 seconds and repeat three times.

3. Leg Circles

Benefits: Improves hip mobility and strengthens the lower abdominals.

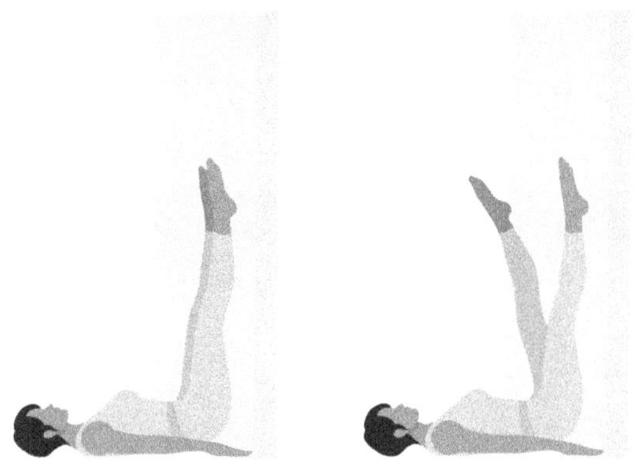

How to Do It: Lie on the floor perpendicular to the wall with both legs up on the wall and move one leg out from the wall and move the ankle in a circle gently, keeping the rest of your body still. Switch legs after a set. Repeat three times.

4. Standing Push-Ups

Benefits: Strengthens the upper body and core.

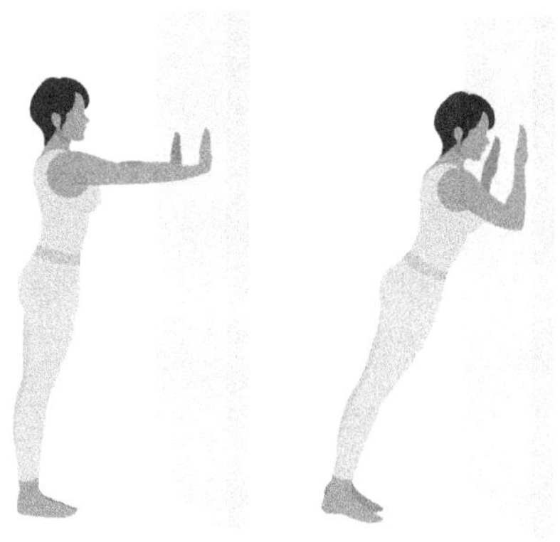

How to Do It: Face the wall, placing your hands flat against it, a bit wider than shoulder-width. Step back so your body forms a diagonal line. Step your feet back. The further your feet are from the wall, the more challenging it will feel. Lower yourself towards the wall, keeping your elbows at a 45-degree angle. Press into the wall to rise back up. Aim for four sets of 10 reps. Rest 30-60 seconds before next exercise.

5. Pelvic Curl

Benefits: Strengthens the lower back and glutes.

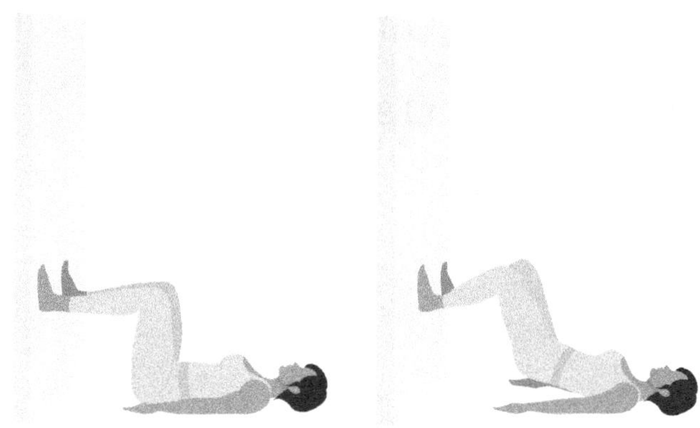

How to Do It: Lie on your back with your feet flat against the wall and knees bent. Lift your hips towards the ceiling, pressing your feet into the wall, and then roll down slowly. Repeat three times.

Rest 30-60 seconds before next exercise.

6. Leg Lift

Benefits: Strengthens your core and back, tones your legs, and improves your balance and stability — vital for both sports and everyday activities. Plus, it increases flexibility and joint motion, keeping you agile as you age.

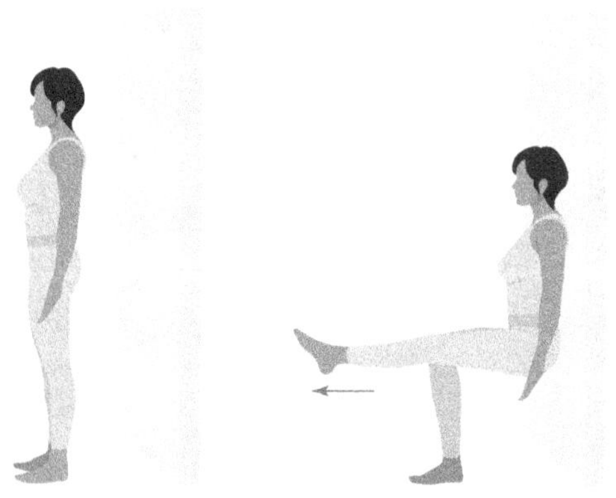

How to Do It: Lean back against a wall with your feet shoulder-width apart, then slide down until your legs form a right angle. Now for the kind of hard part: lift one leg straight out, hold it like a ballet dancer for a slow count of three, and then lower it gently. Switch legs and aim for 10 lifts each. When you're done, just straighten up slowly. Rest 30-60 seconds before next exercise (if it is too hard to do this is squat position, you can modify this one and stand as you lift your leg or just bend your knees slightly).

7. Wall Plank

Benefits: Strengthens the core, shoulders, and arms.

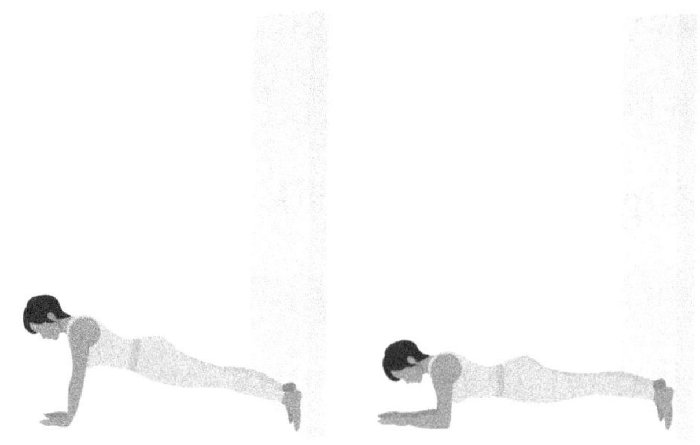

How to Do It: Start in a standing position facing away from the wall. Walk your feet up the wall until your body forms a straight line from head to feet, hands on the ground. Hold this plank position for up to 60 seconds. Repeat three times. You may only start at 30 seconds and then work up to 60 seconds. Rest 30-60 seconds before next exercise (if it is too hard to have your feet on the wall, you can do a regular plank with your feet on the floor and work up to the wall).

8. Glute Leg Lift

Benefits: Strengthen the glutes, enhancing muscle tone and definition. It also improves balance and core stability. Regular practice can lead to better posture and reduced back pain.

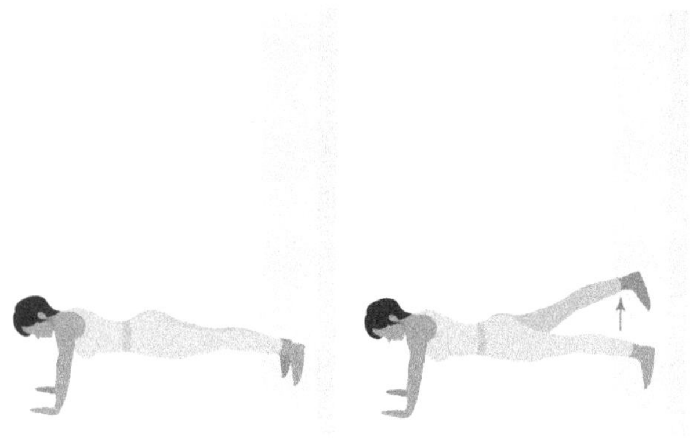

How to do it: Begins by laying down with both feet flat against the wall, move to a plank position and move your feet up the wall so your back is flat. Slowly lift one leg backwards without bending the knee, aiming to get it as high as possible while maintaining balance and keeping your hips square to the floor. Hold the position for a up to 30 seconds before slowly lowering your leg back down to the wall. Alternate legs and aim for 3 repetitions each. Rest 30-60 seconds before next exercise (if it is too hard to keep your feet on the wall, modify by doing starting with a regular plank on the floor).

9. Ab Wall Climbers

Benefits: Strengthens the hamstrings, glutes, and abs.

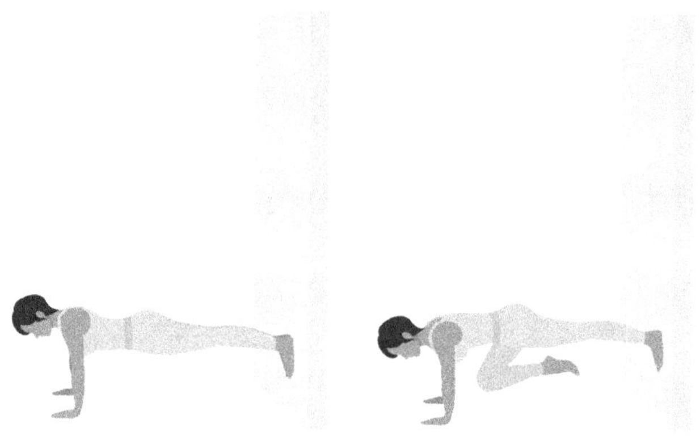

How to Do It: Start in a plank position with your feet against the wall. Keep your abs tight. Lift your leg off the wall, other foot against the wall. Hold for up to 10 seconds. Lower back to the wall slowly. Repeat for 10 reps on each leg. Rest 30-60 seconds before next exercise (if it is too hard with your feet on the wall, try it with your feet on the floor).

10. Calf Raises

Benefits: Strengthens calf muscles and improves ankle stability.

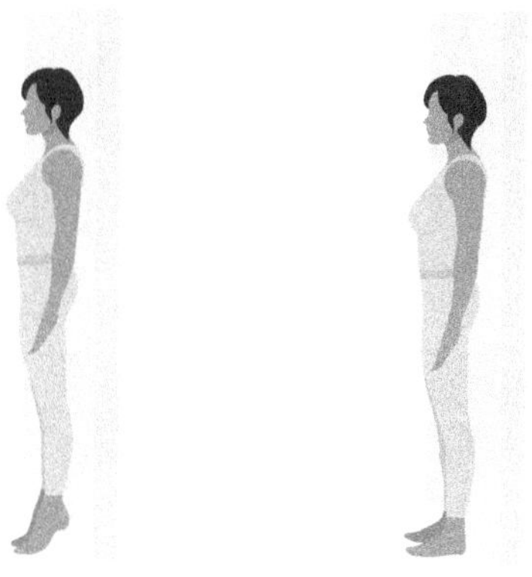

How to Do It: Stand facing the wall with hands on the wall for balance. Lift your heels off the ground, balancing on your toes, then lower back down. For a challenge hold for 30-45 seconds. Repeat three times.

Great Job, you did it! You look Fabulous! Pat yourself on the back! Excellent!

These fabulous exercises are just what you need to kickstart your Pilates journey, darling! They'll help you develop a stunning posture, enhance your flexibility, and sculpt those muscles beautifully. Just remember, breathe deeply and rhythmically as you flow through each movement, and always listen to your body. Take it at your own sweet pace, ensuring it feels right for you. Embrace the journey to a healthier, more vibrant, fabulous you!

Jessica Peters

Conclusion

Embracing Your Inner Radiance with Wall Pilates

Well, my radiant friends, we've reached the end of our journey together, and what a journey it has been! From the first tentative steps into the world of Wall Pilates to the exhilarating moments of strength, flexibility, and mindfulness, you've embraced the magic of movement with grace, courage, and determination.

As you reflect on your journey with Wall Pilates, I want you to take a moment to bask in the glow of your own radiant light. Feel the strength in your body, the peace in your mind, and the love in your heart shining brightly from within. You are a radiant being of light and love, and the world is blessed to have you in it.

But remember, darling, this is just the beginning. Your journey with Wall Pilates is far from over. It's a lifelong adventure, a continuous exploration of your body, mind, and spirit. So, as you step forward into the next chapter of your life, carry with you the lessons you've learned, the strength you've gained, and the love you've cultivated along the way.

And never forget – you are capable of achieving anything you set your mind to. With courage, determination, and a sprinkle of magic, you can move mountains, conquer your fears, and soar to new heights of greatness.

So, my dear, embrace your inner radiance, unleash your limitless potential, and shine your light brightly for all the world to see. The journey may end here, but your light will continue to shine forevermore. Thank you for allowing me to be a part of your incredible journey with Wall Pilates. Your body, mind, and spirit will thank you for it. Let's do this!

Acknowledgments

I would like to express my deepest gratitude to everyone who has contributed to the creation of this book, "Discover Wall Pilates."

First and foremost, I extend my heartfelt appreciation to the dedicated team at Biz Social Marketing, whose expertise and support have been invaluable throughout every stage of the publishing process. Your commitment to excellence and passion for promoting wellness through literature has truly made this project possible.

I am immensely grateful to my health mentors and teachers, whose wisdom, guidance, and inspiration have shaped my understanding of Pilates and its transformative potential. Your dedication to the practice and your unwavering commitment to sharing its benefits with others has been a constant source of motivation and inspiration. Rebecca Walton, I miss the Zoom Yoga and Zoom Zumba we used to do in 2020 and 2021.

I extend my sincere thanks to the individuals who graciously shared their stories, insights, and experiences with wall Pilates, enriching the content of this book and providing real-world examples of its impact on health and wellbeing. Your openness and willingness to contribute have added depth and authenticity to these pages.

Last but not least, I extend my deepest appreciation to the readers of this book. I hope that the practices and teachings shared within these pages will serve as a source of inspiration, empowerment, and transformation on your journey to greater health, vitality, and well-being.

With gratitude,

-Jessica Peters

Jessica Peters

About the Author

Jessica Peters is an accomplished writer and wellness advocate, renowned for her innovative approach to fitness and health. With her latest books, "Discover Chair Yoga" and "Discover Wall Pilates," Jessica has successfully merged her passion for holistic health practices with her keen expertise in accessible fitness solutions. Holding a degree in Health Science, she has dedicated over a decade to promoting physical wellness through various platforms, including workshops and health blogs.

Jessica's expertise shines in her ability to make yoga and Pilates accessible to people of all ages and abilities, emphasizing the importance of integrating gentle yet effective exercises into everyday life. Her work has been featured in prominent health and wellness magazines, establishing her as a trusted voice in the fitness community. Beyond her professional endeavors, Jessica's personal journey with mindfulness and meditation enriches her holistic approach to health, offering readers a deeply personal connection to her teachings.

In her spare time, Jessica enjoys exploring the outdoors and engaging in community wellness events, further reflecting her commitment to a balanced and healthy lifestyle. Her personal and professional experiences make her a relatable and authoritative figure in the world of health and fitness writing.